Practice Progress
How to Maximize
Eye Care
Revenue

Gordon Duncan

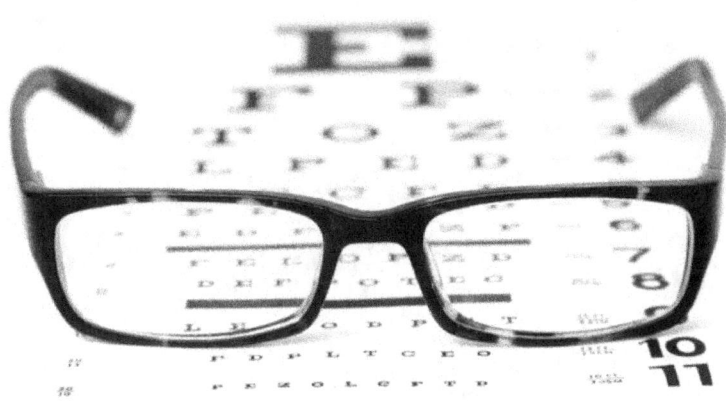

Copyrights

Published in the United States of America

First Edition, 2012

Table of Contents

Copyrights 2

Why You Need This Book 5

Why You Should Listen to Me 6
    Learning to Teach 6
    Making the Sale 7
    Finally, the Eye Industry 7
    Fed Up! - Part One 9
    My Experience with Consultants 10
    Fed Up! - Part 2 11
    What Now? 12
    So What about Me? 13

Necessary Diagnostic Tools 15
    Medical Tools Glossary 16
    Fun with Numbers 17
    MONTHLY TOTALS 18

Now for your work 29
    Projecting in the Middle of the Month 31

Optical – A Black Hole? 34
    Frame Boards – How many frames should we carry? 34
    YOU CANNOT COMPETE WITH WAL-MART 37
    A Word of Warning 40
    YOUR OFFICE IS NOT A CAR LOT 41

Create Cash through Bonuses 44
    Deposit Bonus 44
    Photo Bonus 46
    Insurance Bonus 49
    Optical Bonus 51
    Weekly Bonus 52
    Spiffing Your Front Desk 53

A Simple Effective Marketing Plan 56
    What is the cost? 57

Appendix 58
    Insurance Balance Transfer Policy 59

Patient Pre-Authorization 60

Lost Patient Letter 61

Employee Review 62

One Final Note: 64

Why You Need This Book

Someone once told me that simple is beautiful but simple is never easy. In light of that truth, what I have for you are a few simple practices that will improve your personal practice. They are simple to learn, and once grasped, they are simple to follow. However, they may not be easy at first to implement, but if you are brave enough to make the changes necessary, you will love walking into your practice each day.

This simple toolkit is designed to...

- Give you input, influence, and control in the areas of your practice where presently you have little or none.

- Enable your employees to have ownership so they will motivate themselves to work harder and better.

- Help you make more money in your practice than you ever have before.

Why You Should Listen to Me

A bit of my background will help as you grow in making your practice more efficient and more profitable.

Learning to Teach

Graduating from college, I jumped into the world of education where I taught at-risk youth who had already been expelled from grades 6-12. I was fortunate to be a part of an alternative school that sought to lower the drop-out rate in its system. My first day of teaching was the day the school first opened its doors.

During that time, I was immensely blessed to play a part in changing hundreds of students' lives, and I poured every moment of my day into that goal. I wasn't married yet, so my school day rolled into mentoring which then rolled into evenings of study, grading, and lesson planning.

Simultaneously, I had the great benefit of chairing the English Department, designing curriculum, petitioning the credentialing boards to accept our new school, and all of those responsibilities led me to win the school system's Teacher of the Year. I never imagined that what appeared at first to be a simple teaching job would give me so many experiences to influence, teach, train, administrate, and understand how to lead and manage people.

I ultimately got married and moved an hour away, so I began to look for a new job. My initial intention was to stay in teaching but only if I could continue in the alternate school structure. The county school system that we moved to didn't have one, so I was left with a choice: teach in the old fashion model or find something new to do.

Making the Sale

One day while playing golf, I received a call from a friend of a friend who was looking for an outside salesperson. While sales was not on my radar, the idea of making enough money to pay off my school loans appealed to me. Working with people who I knew and trusted was important to me as well. I quickly became the salesman for a legal document reproduction company. My job was to convince lawyers and paralegals to trust my company with their confidential documents as they prepared for trial.

All of a sudden I was cast into a new world where I was still attempting to influence others, but now that sphere involved efficiency (for my staff), profitability (for my boss), and credibility (for my lawyers). I was in charge of gaining new business and taking care of existing clients. I was daily quoting jobs, making promises (that I had to trust others to keep), and knocking on doors to get appointments.

My years in sales taught me great lessons about patience and persistence. Though I was the face of the organization, I could not act alone, and if my support team didn't trust me, they wouldn't perform.

My company eventually decided to open another office out of state. Unfortunately, that office didn't last a single year. My branch was forced to absorb the costs of the failed branch, and I was left answering questions like, "How long can you go without a paycheck?" My answer was, "I don't work for free."

Finally, the Eye Industry

Perhaps I answered quickly and harshly, but I was not at a place in life where I could just work a month and live without a paycheck. Fortunately, at that same time, an Optometrist friend of mine was in need as his present manager was leaving the workforce to be a full-time mom. After a few meetings, he offered me the job, and I gladly accepted it.

There were some terms of my employment that were key to my taking the job, and as I look back on those things, I can see that my OD did me the biggest favor ever.

In my job, my boss would give me a base salary. He then promised me that he would never give me a raise…ever. However, once I got my legs under me, he would give me 7% of net profit as a bonus. Just for the sake of simplicity. At the end of the month, we looked at how much money we deposited. We would then subtract every penny we spent. If there was anything left over, I got 7% of it.

This was an incredible motivator for me. My doc made it clear: all he wanted to do was come in, turn the dials, and go home. If I was going to be the manager he wanted, then I was going to have to learn and oversee every aspect of the business: front desk, optical, insurance, you name it. If I made those systems work well together, I had the chance to make some real money.

As you can imagine, I cared about every penny, every paperclip, and every patient that walked through the door. We didn't waste anything in that office, and we surely didn't tolerate any one not pulling their weight. Ultimately, I realized that everyone else was going to have to care about the paperclips as well, so I developed a spiff system for the entire office and a specific one for each department. If they cared about the money, then I wouldn't have to worry.

Getting started however, I had to learn the ropes, so I started out by working the front desk for two weeks. I then moved onto pre-testing and optical while my evenings were spent learning how to file insurance and fighting for every dollar. My schooling was quick and overwhelming, but I was soon proficient in each area and my staff learned that I was honest about what I didn't know but confident about what I did. Things rolled along well for several years.

I soon learned that filing insurance for 14,000 patients was too big a job for me to handle in the midst of so many other things, so we farmed it out to a trusted off-site employee. The money spent to file insurance was quickly recouped by the greater % of money that was collected.

Fed Up! - Part One

There were challenges along the way, however. My office was a franchise of a local optometric group. In return for using their software, taking advantage of their discounts, and a few others things, we paid them 4% of billables – that was 4% of what we billed; not 4% of what we collected. I resented writing that check every single month. I just didn't think we received enough benefit for the cost, but that part of the business was a non-negotiable.

Even more annoying to me was the fact that the franchise would send in staff each month to look over our numbers. I will tell you, there is nothing more frustrating than being told how badly you did when you look at numbers that you didn't get to see progress throughout the month. I would be asked why optical sales' averages were dipping or why we didn't see any more patients than we did. Those are difficult questions to answer when you are looking at numbers for the very first time…and they are impossible numbers to change once the month is finished.

My docs would leave those meetings wanting me to do better and work harder. I would leave them frustrated for being the last one in the know.

Ultimately, I made up my mind that I would never go into one of those meetings blindly ever again. I would figure out their systems, determine the numbers myself, and even track them throughout the month so that I could actively affect them. I was done with people yelling at me.

I went home with our monthly numbers printed in detail. I looked at the diagnostics that the franchise honchos cared about and reversed engineered them, and in the process learned their formulas.

I also broke down the prior month's numbers into quarter month increments. I figured out how to project how we were doing with those numbers throughout the month, and I got a better sense for the rhythm of our practice. Next month was going to be different.

As quickly as I learned the numbers and formulas, I taught the staff to do the same. It wasn't going to matter if I cared and they didn't. As they learned how to project and determine the numbers of our days, they grew in working harder towards the things to which they were being held accountable. I soon instituted new financial spiffs for each department. If they hit their numbers, the office hit their numbers, and I hit mine.

I even instituted daily and weekly goals that resulted in food rewards. You won't believe how hard a staff will work for free food. I would say 3-4 out of 5 days, we provided breakfast for the staff and it was common that we would have lunch on a weekly basis. Often, I would spend a mere $15 on muffins to reward the staff keeping the schedule full. It was pennies spent in return for thousands earned.

My Experience with Consultants

Eventually, one of our contact lens companies gave us a national consultant for an entire week. This is back when the government cared a lot less about gifts from vendors. My consultant was very nice. She figured out that working with me instead of working against me was probably the best plan. She dug into all of our numbers, met with me, the staff, and the doctors, and on her last day, she gave us a giant 3 ring binder of recommendations that we should implement.

She hopped onto her plane, flew away, and left my doctors with the expectation that I was to then put into place everything that she recommended. I had very little time to do any of the things she wanted. I soon found out that our contact lens company spent $5,000 to bring her in for the week. I was stunned and frustrated. Our consultant was nice, but all she did was expect me to change a lot of things that I neither signed off on or had the time to put into place.

Fed Up! - Part 2

It was around this time that I started to pursue my Master's degree. My boss told me he didn't care if I took classes as long as it didn't interfere with the profitability of the company. Simultaneously, my doctor sold 51% of the practice to a young OD right out of optometry school. These two decisions (mine and my doctor's) were the beginning of the end for me as a day-to-day manager.

Though my office continued to be profitable at a % consistent with my first few years, I was spending less time at the office. Juggling classes and working was hard. I should have handled the whole situation better, but I rationalized my time away by thinking that as long as profits continued, there would not be a conflict. However, I was not managing our staff as well as I should have been, and my new doctor/owner was not pleased with me at all. He clamped down on my flexible schedule, changed many of the policies, and even proposed changing my bonus structure.

As the majority owner, my new doctor had every right to put whatever policies in place that he wanted. So, he decided to cap my bonuses. He gave me the number and informed that once I received $X amount of bonuses, I wouldn't make any more. Unfortunately, the capping of my bonuses also resulted in the capping of my enthusiasm for my job. Graduate school seemed more and more attractive while the drive to work under the new ownership dimmed. The big questions were:

- What am I going to do?
- If I quit, how am I going to make a living?
- Is it possible to go to school and feed my ever-growing family (My wife was pregnant with our second daughter)?

One day, after a heated exchange with my doc, which I'm sure was as much my fault as his, I drove to make the bank deposit in an absolute funk. I didn't think that I could keep up the miserable existence that was managing the office. I'm sure the doctors wanted me to leave as much as I wanted to leave.

I called my wife that day, and said, "Honey, I think I'm going to put in a 4 month notice today. That will give me time to train someone to take my place and give me time to figure out how we are going to make a living." In an incredible sign of trust, my remarkable wife agreed with me and encouraged me to do just that.

My doctor gladly accepted my offer. That was the easy part. Now, how in the world was I going to keep a roof over my family's house while finishing school?

What Now?

One night, I had a very restless sleep as my brain would not stop thinking about how we were going to make it. When I woke up, it hit me. I might not have had as much experience as our consultant, and I probably couldn't charge $5,000 a week, but I had enough confidence and experience to tackle consulting. Even if I couldn't get five grand a week, I didn't need five grand a week to live. I just had to figure out what I needed to live and find a way to justify that to any doc that would hire me.

My approach was going to have to be a little different than most consultants to convince any doctor to hire an inexperienced contractor like myself. After doing some research about the national guys, I found several niches:

One: I would charge a very economical daily rate – one that wouldn't scare OD's when they heard it.

Two: I wouldn't ask for a contract. If you liked me, ask me back again. If you didn't, we could part company.

Three: I would be willing to help implement any suggestion that I made to a practice. I would either train the staff or actually do the work myself.

My reasoning for these principles was simple: I didn't feel that most consultants justified the large amount of money that they charged. And I didn't think many of them worked very hard. Basically, most national consultants were a big waste of money. From what I could tell, the goal of most consultants was to get as many OD's as possible to sign off on a $1,000 a month (at the least) bank draft with at least a six-month commitment. In return, you might get one full day a month from them and then a lunch phone call or two.

In addition, lots of consultants enjoyed giving advice but never had to be accountable for whether their advice worked or not. They could just blame the results of the ineffectiveness on the staff because the consultants never got their hands dirty. I planned to change all of those things (at least for the doctors with which I worked).

My first paying consulting gig came about when I promised an OD that I would make his good practice better, and if I didn't, he could quickly tell me to go away, no harm, no foul. The risk for the doctor was small, and all the pressure was on me. I jumped in with both feet and began to train staff, make changes, and do whatever it took to help the doc out. If his staff grew in the skills that I was teaching them, and if the practice turned around money-wise, I knew I was doing my job. After six months, that doctor felt that his staff and doctors were properly prepared to take on the future. My time with him was up. Since then, I have had the privilege of working with dozens of OD's and even a few dentists along the way.

So What about Me?

After over 20 years of teaching, selling, managing, and consulting, what I want to do now is empower OD's to improve their practices without having to go broke in the process. Ultimately, if many of the skills in this kit are put into place, most doctors won't need a consultant. They'll gain the managerial tools to accompany their optometric prowess and save a lot of money along the way.

Oh, every now and then, it is helpful to hire an extra pair of eyes, but for the most part, implanting these skills will enable OD's to have a deeper knowledge of their practice, and then they will have skills to put effective plans of change into place.

That is what I want for you. I want you to be able to accurately and objectively assess your practice so that you can make whatever changes you need. I also want you to do that without going broke paying a consultant.

So what follows are some of the tools that I have learned along the way. In each chapter, you'll find not only the formulas necessary to diagnose your practice, but you'll also find helpful examples coupled with suggestions for implementation. When it is all said and done, I want you to feel as confident and as satisfied as you ever have about your practice. Let's jump in.

Necessary Diagnostic Tools

There are countless matrices that you can utilize in diagnosing your practice. This tool kit does not intend to be comprehensive. It does however intend to give you the essential formulas for determining the health of your practice so you can make more money. But as we go forward understand this:

Key Concept - *No number means anything standing alone. Meaning is determined looking backwards and forwards and in relation.*

Let me explain. You may determine a fact about your practice through these formulas. Let's say for example that you find out the total number of comprehensive exams you performed in a month. Maybe that number is 250. Okay, so what? How do you know if that is good or not? Here are sample questions you could ask around that number

- Is that the maximum number of comprehensive exams you can see in one month?

- How many exams did you see last month?

- How many exams did you see in this month last year?

- Is that a healthy number of exams for this time of year?

- Does the upcoming month typically bring in more or less exams?

And I haven't even mentioned contact lens or optical in this equation. Also, as we look at these diagnostic tools, it is going to be important to check them throughout the month and project what the numbers might be if all things stay the same. But I am getting ahead of myself.

For the medical side of your office (we'll get to contacts and optical later), here are a few key tools for you to put into place. I'll go into greater detail of each one and their formulas after the glossary.

Medical Tools Glossary

Monthly Billables (MB)
This number is your total, unadjusted billed dollar amount.

Adjusted Monthly Billables (AMB)
This number is your total billed dollar amount minus your insurance adjustments and write offs.

Write Off Percentage (WO%)
This number is determined by subtracting your Adjusted Monthly Billables (AMB) from your Monthly Billables (MB). That number should then be divided by your Monthly Billables (MB).

Total Exams (TE)
This is the total number of your new and established comprehensive eye exams. No Medical Exams or Intermediate Exams should be listed in this total.

Business Days (BD)
Simply, this is the number of days you were seeing patients in a given month.

Exams Per Day (EPD)
This is the average number of comprehensive exams you see each day. It is your TE divided by your BD.

Occupancy % (OCC%)
This is you're EPD divided by the number of exams that your schedule allows each day.

Deposits (DEP)
This is the total amount money you collected in the month (and hopefully put in the bank).

Price Per Patient (P3)
This is the billable value of each full exam you see in a month. It is your Monthly Billables divided by your Total Exams.

Adjusted Price Per Patient (AP3)

This is the billable value of each full exam you see in a month adjusted. It is your Adjusted Monthly Billables divided by your Total Exams.

Revenue Per Patient (RP2)

This is the money in the bank value of every full exam you see in a month. It is your Deposits divided by Total Exams.

Avg Billable Day (ABD)

This is amount you billed each day that you saw patients. You find this number by dividing your Monthly Billables by Business Days.

Avg Dep Day (ADD)

This is the amount of money you earned for each day you saw patients. You find this number by dividing your Deposits by your Business Days.

Fun with Numbers

Now at this point and time, there are a million other numbers that will help you and we'll get to many of them (especially optical), but we should stop and make some sense out these before moving on. Let me give you some examples of how these numbers can become practically useful.

First of all, several of these numbers should be generated fairly easily, and these require no more complex math than a little simple division. Take a look at your end of month report. Most every practice software can generate this for you.

For the sake of practice, let's say these are the numbers for a 2 OD practice with an optical. The following are numbers that you can determine by simply looking at your end of month report and your scheduling calendar.

MB : $86,547
AMB : $63,568
TE : 301
DEP : $61,432
BD : 20

From these few numbers, you can produce this information.

P3 : MB $86,547 divided by TE 301 = $287
AP3 : AMB $63,568 divided by TE 301 = $211
RP2 : DEP $61,432 divided by TE 301 = $204
ABD : MB $86,547 divided by BD 20 = $4,327
ADD : DEP $61,432 divided by BD 20 = $3,072

Now, none of these numbers will do you any good unless you can apply meaning to them for this specific month. Also, understanding these numbers in the context of the prior month and the corresponding month last year and years prior will be incredibly helpful to you.

So, once we begin to find some meaning here, I would encourage you to go back as far as you can and run these numbers for prior months and years. That way, when you are establishing expectations for yourself and your staff, you will base those expectations off of trends that are specific to your practice and specific to the month in question. Having said that, let's apply some meaning to these numbers. They won't do you any good unless you can find meaning in them.

MONTHLY TOTALS

MB: $86,547 – Is this a good number or a poor number? Well, to begin, remember this is what you billed. You know you will not collect 100% of these monies with insurance involved. One way to determine the health of this number is comparing it to what you billed in the corresponding month last year and the month prior.

Also, it is the rare month where you deposit more than you bill. That only happens when your insurance person has been able to recover outstanding insurance payments. You don't want to be that far behind, but you would be happy when the money came in, but just know that more than likely, you will have deposited less than your MB. Having said that, here are a few questions to help you determine the health of your MB.

- Did your MB rise or fall compared to the same month last year?

- Did your MB rise or fall compared to last month?

- Knowing what you need to deposit each month to pay your bills, is this a strong enough number to get you to that desired deposit?

Obviously, lots of things affect what you bill including TE's, optical, contact lens sales, etc. When you see your MB rise or fall, either for the month or according to your expectations, you can then seek out those individual numbers (and we'll talk about how to do that later) to determine how they affected your MB.

AMB: $63,568 and WO% 26% – These two numbers really have to be taken together. Your adjusted monthly billable is your total dollar amount billed minus your adjustments. More than likely, you will always have some amount of money to write-off. These write-offs should come in one of two forms. You will write off the difference between what you bill for a certain procedure and the amount you agreed to accept from any insurance company in which you have a relationship. And you can also have write-offs from uncollectable insurance or patient balances.

So is an AMB of $63,568 a healthy number or not? That depends on the WO%. This WO% is 26% and is pretty high. At this point and time, you are giving away $.25 of every dollar you bill or essentially giving away $1 out of every $4. What is a healthy number? That's hard to say because it will depend on what insurance contracts you have signed.

You may find upon examination that some of them just aren't worth the effort if even after collecting co-pays, you are still writing off tons of money.

Insurances being a necessary evil for most, there are three primary culprits (aside from insurance) that can cause your write-offs to soar.

1. Billing patients for fees that they don't agree to pay

2. Failure to collect money due at check out

3. The lack of a proper follow up system with patients who owe you money.

Let's talk about each of these for a moment. You might say, "Well who bills a patient for something in which the patient doesn't agree to pay?" It happens all the time. Many doctors leave the discussion of contact lens fitting fees to their techs, and the tech doesn't like to talk about money. Many times patients don't understand that those fees are more than likely not covered by insurance. Routine examination photos are typically not covered by insurance. Does your patient understand that? Basically, examine your procedures, and then ask yourself these questions:

- Does every patient understand that all co-pays are due at time of service?

- Is there a system in place to explain contact lens' fees to patients?

- Do your patients understand that they can neither order contacts nor receive a copy of their prescription unless they have paid for the contact lens services?

- Does your front desk have a zero tolerance policy in terms of allowing patients to leave with outstanding balances?

- Do you let patients schedule new services or order new product if they have an outstanding balance? You shouldn't.

- Do you have an accountability system for the employees who check out patients and allow them to leave balances unpaid?

One of the more challenging aspects of keeping your WO% down is a proper system to collect outstanding balances. When I was the primary insurance collector of my office, I had a monthly meeting with my OD's about our receivables. They expected no more than 3% of our insurance A/R to be in the 60 days or older category. Any amount of money I wrote off that was 60 days or older had to be justified before the OD's. These same policies were applied to patient receivables as well.

In light of those facts, I had a rigorous system in place. Bills went out promptly to patients on the first of every month. Each current bill went out as is. Anything 30 days or older included a personal note and then a follow up phone call before the account reached 60 days. At 60 days, patients were warned of impending collections via letter and a phone call. At 90, patients were turned over to collections.

Outstanding insurances were treated with equal vigorism. A competent insurance person will re-file or transfer proper balances within 1-2 days of receiving EOB's. Over 60's will be kept under 3% of total, and no write offs in the over 60 category are to be done without justification.

Honestly, I've seen practices that could zero out their entire debt load only if they trimmed their receivables totals. This is no easy job, and it requires an employee who enjoys the hunt. A good insurance person should be rewarded as well, but we will take that up in our chapter of spiffs. As for now, a 25% WO% is high and should be pursued.

Now, before heading onto the next number, consider this. Some of you may have a policy in place where patients can pay a portion of their contact lens or optical orders at the time of service with the agreement that they will pay the balance at pick up.

Whatever number you choose should be adhered to religiously. I honestly don't recommend a pay down system for contacts, but if you do, nothing less than 50% should be paid up front. That number covers your cost at least. Then, if the patient fails to pick up the contacts, you can return them at no cost to the practice. I recommend at least 50% for optical as well. However, cut lens can't be returned as easily.

Explain to patients that they must pay 50% for glasses up front, and if they do not pick them up, they will have to pay a restocking fee of some sort. But most importantly, never, and I mean never, should any product be picked up without payment in full. That is practically giving money away and is the quick plan towards crazy, outstanding receivables.

Listen, let's be honest. It will be a temptation for every insurance/billables collector to write off some fees that they know that they can't or will have a hard time to collect. It is up to you to pay attention to these numbers every month. A scheduled accountability meeting must be in place.

TE: 301 – Is 301 a good number of exams? That depends on lots of things. One aspect to consider is finding out what you did last year during the same month. It is essential that a practice track how many full exams they see each month. A practice has to learn their own rhythm and manage their expectations accordingly.

For example, I used to consult with an OD whose entire city would practically shut down in the middle of a certain month for the town's furniture market. Hitting a high number of exams that month was always a challenge. Knowing that ahead of time allowed the OD to wisely plan for either personal time off or employee time off. Avoiding excess expenses around that time was also wise. But planning on higher than average number of exams the next month was part of their expectation as well after tracking these numbers.

But more importantly, how does that TE compare with the maximum possible of exams you can have each day and month?

Every practice should have a scheduling template that informs them how many exams they can see in a day. Some OD's are built for a full exam every 15 mins while some need 20 or 30. Installing a template is absolutely essential for seeing the maximum possible exams, and it is also essential to train staff how to schedule.

Making that template is really about understanding your community need, your office capacity, and your own work desire. I know several practices that schedule sick eyes and follow ups at the beginning and end of each shift. Meaning, they have 30 mins set aside for 3 appointments at the beginning of the day, right before lunch, right after lunch, and right before the close of business. That way, apart from emergencies, the majority of your day is given over to comprehensive exams.

There is nothing more frustrating that working hard all day seeing patients and then you realize that the majority of your day was given over to non-revenue generating procedures due to poor scheduling. Contact lens follow ups and the like are important, but they should be scheduled in such a way as to free up an OD to see the maximum number of comprehensive exams each day.

Many ODs that I speak to are frustrated with cash flow issues. They'll say, "I work hard all day every day." And though that might be true, many times those ODs are killing themselves with an unorganized scheduled that maximized their time but minimizes their profits.

Billable Days (BD): 20 – This is perhaps the simplest data that you can collect, but it will add incredible meaning to your numbers. Simply, how many days did you see patients? Depending upon whether you work Saturdays or not, this number for a practice with a full-time OD is somewhere between 18-24.

Sometimes, OD's have a hard time figuring out why their numbers are low. But if you have a holiday or two in a month, your BD's might be down. There is no need to yell at your staff if your numbers are low if you have less BD's. You can't bill if you don't see patients.

As for offices with multiple OD's, each doctor's day is a billable day. Two full-time OD's seeing patients all day, every day for a month is 40 BD's give or take. If your doc takes off at lunch on Friday, that is a half day. Knowing your BD's ahead of time will play a part when we start projecting our numbers mid-month, but we aren't quite there yet.

Exams per Day (EPD): 15.05 – 301 comprehensive exams divided by 20 business days is 15.05 exams per day. Is this a good number? It all depends on how your schedule is set. If you want to see 4 an hour with follow ups and sick eyes at the beginning and end of each morning and afternoon, you can conceivably see 24+ exams a day.

Occupancy % (OCC%): 75% This office was set for 24 exams a day, so dividing your EPD by the OCC% and you discover that this office's schedule is 75% filled.

Deposits (DEP): $61,432 - Well, the truest determination for the health of your deposits is whether or not this number covers your bills, your payroll, your liabilities, and even better, leaves some money left over at the end of the month. It may seem silly, but if you are monitoring all of the above but not tracking deposits, more than likely, you are leaving money on the table. Towards that end, let's look a few things to monitor about your deposits.

It is absolutely essential that you know what your "nut" is each month. Your nut is your essential operating expenses. This is every bill, payroll, every minimum on a credit card, every liability payment, and anything else that you have to pay to remain current on your bills. If you don't take a salary, figure out what it should be and add it up. If you are not paying all your minimums, figure it out and add it up.

Determine your nut so you can know what your basic goal must be each month. Don't practice blind, and don't assume the numbers will take care of themselves. They won't. Figure out your nut, and set your goals on it and beyond.

I know this is a discussion of income and not expenses, but allow me one moment to speak to expenses. I once worked for a doctor who treated the office bank account like a personal atm. As an owner, he had that right. He could take any amount out that he wanted and categorize it as an owner's distribution. But because of that habit, he rarely had enough money in the bank to pay his bills. As his bookkeeper, I was so frustrated. I always encouraged him to figure out his salary needs and take it so the office could plan accordingly.

It won't matter how much money you put in the bank if you choose to just take money out at will for salary or for fun.

Lunches can work the same way. You have the right for the company to pay for your lunches if you want. But if you are not covering your expenses, pack a lunch and take care of your company. I have also seen offices struggle for the simple fact that the docs just refuse to quit spending $25 a day on lunch (or $6,500 a year).

Price Per Patient (P3): $287 – What in the world is this? Essentially, your P3 is the billable value for each full exam you see. I'm sure that there are other names for this, but P3 came up for me years ago in my practice and it just stuck. What is the price (value) billed every time you see a full exam? Once you determine that number, the hard part is to figure out whether that number is healthy or not.

Your P3 takes in every single dollar that your office bills. It includes every exam, contact lens fee, office visit, and yes, your optical and contact lens orders. Even though a host of factors influence your P3, the viability of your practice still comes down to how many exams you see. So your MB divided by your TE's gives you the best sense of value. Obviously, you want your optical and contact lens efforts to be incredibly high, as that will help, but for now, let's just focus on P3.

There are a couple of things to remind yourself about your P3. Having a higher P3 is not better unless you can collect it. Who cares if your P3 is $543 a patient if you write off 50% of that number and your deposits are low? Then you are just wasting time billing things that you can't collect. High P3's only matter if your deposits are high as well. High billables must correlate to low write offs and high deposits.

Take this in mind when you price your optical. If you are writing off $200 every time you sell a frame, you probably should adjust your prices accordingly. If you have a habit of telling patients that you'll be glad to file visits to their insurance and they can pay later if the claim is denied, you are going to have low deposits and will more than likely write a good bit of your billables off.

So what is a healthy P3? National average is reported all over the place from $275 to $325, so $300 is a good number. If you are above that number, rejoice, but make sure your AMB is not too far away from your P3 and make sure your deposits are high. If you are P3 is below $300, ask yourself if you or your staff are aggressive enough in filling the schedule, selling contacts, and selling glasses.

Adjusted Price Per Patient (AP3): $211 – Well as you can imagine by now, your AP3 is your Adjusted Monthly Billables divided by your Total Exams. The % difference between your MB and your AMB will be the exact same as the difference between your P3 and your AP3. This dollar amount is your true billable value of each comprehensive exam.

Revenue per Patient (RP2): $204 – Once again, the numbers get more and more critical. Your RP2 is determined by your Dep divided by TE's. Why does this number matter? When you know it, you can know the exact dollar amount that goes in the bank every time you see a full exam. Once you know it, other things become incredibly important. One more exam equals another $204.

You ask yourself. "How can I increase this number without sacrificing patient care?" You care a lot more when there is an open slot that isn't filled. You care a lot more when you weigh closing the office for a day or a half day. You care a lot more when you count how many business days there are in a month. RP2 tells you, "My practice grows by this dollar amount every time we gain a new patient."

Knowing this number is so helpful when you decide to make new purchases for your practice, consider adding staff, or even hiring a new OD. Once you know the cost of an additional expenditure or its monthly cost, you can simply compute the number of new exams a month you need to add to cover that cost.

For example, if you are going to take on a new server for your office computers, and you know you are going to wind up spending $932 a month, and you also know that your revenue per patient is $204 a month on average, it doesn't take a rocket scientist to figure out what you have to do. You need to increase your number exams per month by 4.5.

Over Head Average (OHA): Now this number hasn't come up before, so let me explain what it is. This company needs $74,032 a month to pay all its bills. You divide your RP2 into your monthly overhead and you get your OHA. This office needs 363 to pay its bills. This office needs 363 exams before it banks a single dollar.

On a side note, discovering this for yourself is going to take some extra work on your part and might involve some help from your accountant. Do this: find out what your average monthly expenses are. Not what you want them to be, but find out what you average spending each month. Get that number and learn it and know it. Then do the math. I know it might scare you a bit, but do it. Divide that number by your RP2. You know what you get? You get your OHA. You will find out the number exams you have to see each month to make payroll, pay your rent/lease, and put food on your table.

Does that number scare you or reassure you? Either way, you now know your nut.

Once you determine your number (or at least what your average is over the course of a year), you can rest easy each month once you pass the minimum you need to cover your overhead).

ABD: $4,327 and ADD: $3,072 – By dividing the company's Monthly Billables (MB) and their DEP by the Business Days (BD), they see what they bill each day and what they deposit each day. Again, knowing this number will make any company reckon well how many days they are closed per year.

Now for your work

So there we have it. We are going to cover a lot more numbers, but those are your basics. Don't worry, your optical and other areas are coming up, but those are your most important numbers. Every single month you need to know them. In fact, go backwards and map as far as you have good data. Map out the stats for every single month you have ever been opened for business if you can.

Let's have you give it a shot. Get the last month's numbers and do the hard math. Figure it out for yourself before you let the spreadsheet do it for you. Try to find your last month's numbers for these categories:

MB:
AMB:
WO%
TE:
BD:
EPD:
OCC%:
DEP:
P3:
AP3:
RP2:
ABD:
ADD

What did you discover? Ask yourself the following questions to help you determine some next steps.

MB

- Did you bill as much as you expected during this month?
- Was your MB even above your OHA?

AMB and WO%

- Was your AMB and WO% higher and lower than you expected?
- If it was higher than expected, what steps do you need to do find out why so much was written? Remember, your WO% does not rise because you received insurance money.
- Your %'s will always be the agreed upon amount from your insurance companies. An exorbitant WO% means that some amount of money was unrecoverable and was written off.
- Find out what that was and get someone to justify it.

TE, BD, EPD, and OCC%

- Did you see as many TE's as it felt like you did?
- Are your BD's representative of a typical month for you?
- Was this a month when you had an abnormal number of days without patients (November, December, Vacation Month, etc)?
- How did those number of days affect your MB and DEP?
- Were your EPD even close to what your template allotted?
- Do you have someone who responsible for the schedule? Ask that staff person to print the schedule 3 random days from the last month. Check and see how close it was to the template. Manage accordingly.

DEP

- No one is ever pleased with their deposits, but does this number cover your expenses?
- Is it equivalent to the work and effort you put in this month?
- Knowing what you need to pay your bills, are you presently banking money or losing money?
- If you are losing, is it already so serious that you need to consider cutting costs? If so, what might those costs be?

P3 and AP3

- The % difference between your P3 and your AP3 should be the same difference between your MB and your AMB.
- Looking at what you billable value is for each full exam, begin to think about you can do to increase that number without causing your AP3 to rise. We'll pursue this more as we look at your optical and other numbers.

RP2

- This is the money you put in the bank every time you saw a patient.
- Check your accounts receivables. Is your "present" field full of $10 and $25? Then people aren't collecting copays.
- What is your standard contact lens exam cost when an existing patient has no change? Let's say it is $40. Look for $40 on your accounts receivable. Speak to your staff if you find any. No one should leave while owing money, and be sure to check that those patients with balances didn't order and receive contacts.

ABD and ADD

- It's good to know these numbers. Affect all the numbers above and you will see an effect in ABD and ADD.
- You can only increase it if you bill more and collect more. Just being open won't affect it unless you have a backlog of patients you are trying to accommodate.

Projecting in the Middle of the Month

When I was a manager and the big wigs from the franchise would show up at the end of the month to bust me up for not hitting the numbers, I eventually just got fed up. What good was it for me to know the numbers after the numbers were sealed, put in a coffin, and buried in the ground? Like I said, that is how I came up with the diagnostics above, but that wasn't good enough. I had to be able to manipulate those numbers before they made it into the ground.

That's where projecting comes into play. And here is the good thing: it is really easy.

First of all, always know how many business days you have each month. For the sake of example, our practice is going to have 21 this month. Hurray, that's a good month. Along the way, you should stop at the end of given business day and project how you are going to do that month. I was obsessive. I would do it every day, but that is not necessary. I suggest doing it at least 4 times a month. Let's give it a shot.

Below are sample numbers 7 days into the month. Beside it are the average numbers per day so far, and beside that are the projected numbers for the month.

	Month to Date	Average for 7 Days	Projected Totals
MB:	$26,743	$3,820	$80,228
AMB:	$21,394	$3,056	$64,182
WO%	20%	20%	20%
TE:	83	11.86	249
DEP:	$24,554	$3,508	$73,662
P3:	$322	$322	$322
AP3:	$258	$258	$258
RP2:	$296	$296	$296

Whether these projected numbers are encouraging or not depends upon a lot of factors. But you get the point. Just as I learned when I was meeting the franchise big wigs, you can't change a number unless you know what it is ahead of time. Projecting gives you the ability to know where your month is trending, but more importantly, projecting gives you the time to put whatever changes are needed in place before it is too late.

You might ask, "How in the world am I going to change any of these things? The numbers are the numbers." Well, there is nothing any consultant can tell you to immediately add one patient to practice. However, there are ways to motivate your staff to go find that patent and to better serve them when they are in your office.

The picture here is spiffing or incentivizing your staff. But before we jump into that, let's make a few things clear.

- You can't change and outcome unless you know where it is trending.

- Neglecting regular projections is a refusal to manage your staff and care for you practice.

- Figuring out what motivates your staff is key.

But before we jump in there, let's look at a few more key diagnostics in the other areas of practice. That way, we can talk about spiffing each employee and each area of your office.

Optical – A Black Hole?

The one place that many practices allow money to just disappear is their optical. It should be the other way around. The one place that practices should make a ton of money is in their optical. As I have visited offices, I've come to realize that many OD's entrust their optical to other employees, and what happens is that an accepted ignorance sets into their thinking. It is almost like the doc thinks that he/she doesn't have enough time to oversee the optical. Hopefully, you have an outstanding optician/frame seller, but no matter the talent or level of managerial skill, the optical has got to be looked after vigorously.

The problem that I see most docs face is knowing where to start. There isn't one magic spot, so let's just walk through areas in which your management can have a quick and profitable impact. Let's do that by asking a series of questions.

Frame Boards – How many frames should we carry?

This truly is a difficult question, but if you don't answer it, either your frame buyer or a frame seller will answer it for you. I know a few practices that carried massive amounts of debt because their frame buyer just got out of control. Remember: you are the final frame buyer. I don't care how great your seller/optician is, give them a financial limit. Tell them they have the freedom to buy frames to a certain dollar amount or to a certain number, but any potential purchase that exceeds those amounts has to be approved by you.

I used to tell my optical folks this next truth all the time, but they always struggled to believe it. The frame seller is not your friend. What I mean is that they are not your personal friend. Oh, they might take you out to eat, and I've even known a few to show up at birthday parties and the like, but the end goal of that frame seller is to make the sale.

I've seen offices that gave frame sellers nearly 100% freedom to bring in frames, which is insane. If you give a salesperson unrestrained freedom, what you are going to get is an unrestrained frame bill. And don't let the seller fool you with the old "I'm just going to swap out some frames" routine. If you don't know what I'm talking about, let me explain.

Your optical person tells the frame seller that you won't be buying any new frames from them this visit. They respond with, "Hey, no problem. Everyone is tightening up right now. I'll help you and take some of these old frames that aren't selling and just put some new one out to help boost your sales. We'll just swap out the old ones for new ones." Then guess what happens? You get a bill for $500.

I'm not impugning every seller. Some of them have amazing integrity, but their job is to make the sale. They make more money the more frames that they sell. Whenever a seller wants to "swap out" here are is the simple rule. Tell them that if they want to take away frames that aren't selling and replace them with newer frames, that is great. But in the end, the effect on your account must either be that I have a credit for returned frames or the swap out costs me nothing. Period. Any seller that violates this rule or this trust will be placed on probation or banned. It may sound harsh, but no seller has your interests first. Only you do.

Once I put this rule in place, I faced a ton of opposition from my optical staff. They said our sellers were honest and that it would damage our relationships with them if we started talking to them that way. I asked them what some of our sellers had done for them lately in terms of gifts and meals. They listed a string of gifts. That was the real problem. They didn't want to lose all their freebies, but the problem was that their freebies came at a cost of thousands to the office.

Do not be swayed on this. What you'll find with this approach is that you'll be offered a lot less swapping deals, but if you do, you'll get new frames at no additional cost. Implement this policy now. Do not be dissuaded by your optical staff.

If you don't manage or restrain your optical folks from buying, you are going to wind up with a ton of understock. Understock is that stash of frames you keep in a cabinet or in the back or maybe even in boxes in the attic (believe me when I say I have seen this).

I once worked with an office that was the largest in a very small town. They were the kings of the roost and the big fish in a small pond if you will. Their office also posted a loss or barely broke even most months. Figuring out why was my job. Actually, my job was to increase revenue, but what I learned was their revenue was great (I know; you can always have more). Their problem was their astronomical frame bills. I learned that if they could reduce their frame bills even by just 25%, they would be profitable again.

The doc just couldn't understand why his frame bills were so high, so I had to figure out what was going on in optical. What I discovered was shocking to the doc. He had nearly 800 frames in understock, and his sellers just kept buying more. And most of the frames under the boards were junk.

It looked like the OD had completely entrusted the frame buying to his optician, and she just kept buying and buying. Granted, the stuff she had on the board looked great, but it came at the expense of a ton of understock and some outrageous bills. Since she didn't pay the bills, and since she didn't have a sense of the office's finances, she assumed everything was okay. It was a hard day of reckoning for everybody.

So, back to our original question: how many frames should you carry on your frame board? I would suggest whatever you can turn over 2.5 times a year. If you sell 1,000 frames a year (God bless you by the way), then you need 400 frames on your board. Along the way, you don't really need any more than bout 50 frames in understock. If your attempt is to carry every size and every color of every frame, then you are going to go broke, so don't try to do it.

There is another distinct advantage to carrying the number of frames that you can turn over 2.5 times (in addition to the cost savings). That number of frames keeps the patient from being overwhelmed, and an overwhelmed patient goes elsewhere. Let me explain.

When you go to a car dealer, they set the cars up in an attractive way to get your attention. You'll find a couple of high end, exclusive cars in the showroom. A few other cars will be in prominent display out in front. You might find 2-3 rows of cars on each side, and not much else. Now, there are ton more cars out back, but everything is set out in such a way that the buyer is not overwhelmed. If you want a certain color or a certain option, they go and find the car for you on the lot or call another dealership in town. But what you see is just enough to entice you.

Though this is an imperfect analogy, I think you see where I'm going. If you sell a 1,000 frames a year and they are all on the board, the patient can't see the forest for the trees. The dealer doesn't put every car they are going to sell on the lot at the same time and they strategically place the ones available just in sight.

Even Wal-Mart opticals don't put every frame out. They have a ton of understock because they can afford it, but they are very specific and choosy about what makes it onto the board. Everything at one time is just too much.

So don't put a ton of frames on your board. Too many options equals too many decisions which just might result in no sale for you.

Speaking of Wal-Mart. Let me give you another bit of advice about stocking your board. Say this next bit of advice out loud if you have to or write it on your bathroom mirror. Order fortune cookies with it if that is what it takes to get this advice into your head and heart.

YOU CANNOT COMPETE WITH WAL-MART

Here is what I mean. If you think $79 for a full set of glasses or making your living off of cheap "Buy one; get one free" offers is going to help you compete against the world's 25th largest national economy, then you are fooling yourself. Wal-Mart could pay every independent OD's patients to leave their practices, give them a set of frames in their store, and still make money. So, when you choose to stock your board, you have to take a couple of approaches.

First of all, you don't have to be a boutique ($300 frames and up only), but if you can be, go for it. If not, act like one. Let me explain. If you try to make a living in the buy one get one free world, you lose the right to be critical of massive chains. You can't point out their quite often inferior quality if you are doing the exact same thing. They can at least afford to replace junk frames that break, and you can't. Aim higher.

If someone asks you if you have special deals or $79 full sets, offer this advice to them. "While I respect my other OD's who work at Wal-Mart, the reason those frames are so cheap is because they are inferior quality. I never want one of my patients to walk out the door only to have them return a month later with frames that fell apart in their hands."

In terms of the economy, address it in this way. "I know that paying a couple of hundred dollars for a pair of glasses is not easy these days. But what is even worse is spending money on an inferior pair of glasses that is going to waste your time and cause you to make multiple trips to Wal-Mart. And you know what that optician is going to do? They'll offer to replace it no problem, and then they'll suggest you walk around Wal-Mart in the meantime. You'll get another set of junk glasses, and you can pick them up right after you spend $100 in the super store."

I'm not joking. Be that honest. Sell quality frames and make no excuses for either their cost or their quality. Trust me on this. I would rather go broke selling quality materials than go broke replacing junk frames and having really expensive employees waste time doing the same thing over and over again.

Sell quality. Sell service. Sell what you can offer that they can't: personal service that is second to none.

So what do you charge for your frames? Well, here is what most docs do. They have a set mark up for their frames. I know some that double and some that triple their frame cost. I recommend tripling, but look at your market and make your determination. But don't stop there. If all you do is triple your frame cost, then you have a million different prices on your board. That doesn't help sales. Let me explain.

When a patient looks at your board and they find every frame has a different price, two things stick in their mind: the highest and lowest price. The highest price is probably beyond their budget, so their mind settles on the lower number. Let's say that number is $99. They are going to go cheapest, but they are probably going to stay somewhere around that number. So what do you do?

The answer is set price points and stick to them in your optical. Here is the concept. Set your cheapest frame price. I would suggest $99, but if you feel like you have to go to $79, do that. Then set your highest frame price say at $399. Then determine 5 prices in between that are equal amounts apart. For example, your board prices would look like this.

$99, $159, $219, $279, $339, and $399

Some folks like to go away with all their frames ending in 9, but that is probably neither here nor there. The idea with price points works like this. You want repetitive prices sticking in your patient's head. When they see the same number come up again and again, most patients will kick out the highest and lowest and settle on a good number in between. If you have 400 frames and 400 frame prices, the patient's mind sticks to the highest and the lowest.

So when you get your frames in, pricing is easy. The formula will look like this. And again, I'll use the 3x's mark up as our example.

Frame Cost x 3 rounded up the closest price point.

So, if you buy a lot of frames for $66 dollars, then this is how you will price them. $66 x 3 = $198. Then you round it up to $219. If you get frames at a special rate, still use the standard frame cost for that frame. So if you buy lot of frames that are typically $99 at the price of $79, use the $99 cost. $99 frames x 3 = $297. You'll round those frames up to $339.

Now let me go ahead and warn you. If you tell your frame staff that they have to reprice, retag, and rescan all of their frames, they are not going to be happy. If you explain to them that it will increase their sales (that is if you spiff them on sales), they'll be okay with it in the long run. If you don't spiff your sellers, then you are just going to have to tell them this is the way it is.

In the end, you may decide that price points are not the way to go. That's fine, but I will encourage you to resist an infinite number of frame prices. I even know docs that resist prices that end in 9. No matter what, just make the pricing of your frames strategic. If this system doesn't work, fine. Either find another or create your own, but don't let that revenue stream go un-shepherded.

A Word of Warning

Now, how many price points you want, where you start, and where you stop are ultimately decisions that you need to make for your practice in light of your location and the local economy. Once you set these prices, your sellers will eventually grow comfortable with the idea if you manage them well. Please guard against this one possible effort to subvert your new plans. Do not let your sellers barter with their frames and lens.

I've been in offices that felt like flea markets because the frame sellers were negotiating every single cost to the patient. I know that some folks feel this gives them the opportunity to compete with Wal-Mart, but it doesn't. All individual bargaining does is make you and your practice look cheap.

YOUR OFFICE IS NOT A CAR LOT

People feel comfortable brokering deals at car lots because they know that the sticker price is not the price that the owners will accept. Buyers know that the sticker prices are a jacked up price with some fluff built in, so counter offers are expected. Don't let your optical fall into this trap.

If your frame seller's chief tool for closing a sale is to instantly drop the price, then instantly drop the frame seller. You don't need them. Have you ever wondered what goes through the mind of a patient when a frame deal is being brokered? Maybe you didn't even know this happens in your office, but I bet it does. So, back to the question: what goes through the patient's mind when all of a sudden, your frame seller says, "Tell you what, if it will help, I can take 20% off these frames." Yes, I'm sure the patient is thankful and maybe even enticed, but what goes through their head is, "I knew these frames were overpriced." I even heard a seller one time say, "Listen, the doctor sets these prices, and I know they are expensive, so I tell you what, I can give you a 20% discount right now." If anything like that ever comes out of one of your employee's mouth, fire them on the spot. You don't need them.

Bartering means you charge too much. Instead, here is a better option. For patients with optical insurance benefits, give them what they plan dictates. If it is $105 towards frames, great give it to them. If it is 30% off, great give it to them. But then tell your patients that Hipaa compliance won't allow you to deviate from the patient's plan to cut a special deal (which is true). If you want to make it a practice to give a standard 20% off for every patient that doesn't have any optical benefits, great. Do that, but stick to just that. But bottom line it for your patients (and especially the seller who wants to barter), brokering individual deals with patients violates the Hippa principle of every patient being treated the same. Don't let anyone or anything endanger your practice in such a way, especially a lazy seller who wants to cut an individual deal with each and every patient.

One last thing before we move into some of the practical numbers that you need to look for each month. If a person is dead set on buying cheap frames from giant box store, there is very little you can do about it. But this one thing is always true: it is in the patient's best interest to purchase frames and lens from the practice in which they received their eye exam.

Selling this point to your patient is first and foremost your responsibility. I know some docs don't prefer to talk prices or frames sales at all, and I get that, but you must make every effort explain to your patient the inherent value of buying frames from you. Here are a few suggestions.

First of all, new frames and lens should be a part of your examination. Of course, I would never encourage you to push new lenses on a patient who doesn't need them, but if you can't express the need for different frames for different purposes or the ocular health benefits of UV coating, don't expect anywhere else to either.

If a patient doesn't need frames, take notice as to whether they have an optical benefit or not. Encourage them not to let that benefit go to waste. Encourage them in this way.

"Ms X, you don't really need new lenses this year. Your prescription hasn't changed that much. But you do have a frame and lens benefit from your insurance company. Those benefits are yours and you paid for them. They just go away if you don't use them. Ask our gal over in optical if she can help you find a pair that won't cost you too much. You might find a relatively inexpensive pair and get them tinted for sunglasses."

Second, walk your patients to optical if you can. This is where you most often learn that a patient is planning on shopping at the big box store. Again, it is up to you.

"You know, Ms X, I don't blame you for checking out Giant Store on the Corner. We had a cookout recently, and it made plenty of sense to buy everything from there. But buying a box of 24 frozen hamburger patties and buying a pair of glasses are two completely

different things. Granted, they are probably cheaper than us. They buy entire freighters of frames at a time whereas we buy a dozen. But when you get your glasses from us, you can trust that the relationship between me and you is met well by our folks over in optical. They can ask me questions that the seller over at Wal-Mart can't ask me. And if you have any problems, you receive my personal guarantee that you will be satisfied."

The most advantage edge that you have over the big box store is you. You can out quality, out serve, and out care them any day. What you can't do is go toe to toe with prices. They will win that battle every single time.

Now as you assess the health of your optical, consider paying attention to these numbers every month.

Optical numbers

Frames sold – This is the total number of frames you sell each month.

Frames average – This is the average cost of the frames you sold.

Frames % - This is the percentage of your comprehensive exams that purchased frames or frames sold divided by full exams.

I know that many of you are going to struggle with this next concept, but hear me out. You have got to spiff your employees. I'm sure you pay them a fair salary, maybe even an above-average salary, but most employees will go above and beyond for some extra cash/benefits. The way for you not to go broke giving those spiffs is by basing all of them on improvement and efforts above and beyond.

Let me give you a few examples, not only for your optical but for your whole house.

Create Cash through Bonuses

Deposit Bonus

This is an all staff bonus that directly helps you put money in your pocket while motivating your staff. Here is how it works.

- Create a 12 month chart from the prior year that lists what your deposits were for each month
- Then project 5, 10, 15, and 20% growth.
- Affix a value for each employee if they meet this goal.

Before I show you an example, let me address a few fears. You may not want your employees to know your deposits, but I will say they already do. They have a sense of how money your office takes in, and it is probably an overly-skewed sense. Go ahead and tell them the truth. For most of them, it will be a reality check.

Secondly, don't worry about paying out these bonuses. You only have to pay them out when your office improves its deposits from last year and the payout for most offices is only a tiny % of the extra money you have put in the bank. Let me demonstrate for you.

Deposit Goals – 20xx

Last Yr.	Dep	5% ($100)	10% ($125)	15% ($150)	20% ($175)
Jan	66,327	69,643	72,960	76,276	79,592
Feb	71,754	75,342	78,929	82,517	86,105
Mar	80,858	84,901	88,944	92,987	97,030
April	87,763	92,151	96,539	101,042	105,316
May	77,089	80,943	84,798	88,652	92,507
June	80,223	84,234	88,256	92,256	96,268
July	71,673	75,257	78,840	82,424	86,008
Aug	75,674	79,458	83,241	87,025	90,809
Sep	76,026	79,827	83,629	87,430	91,231
Oct	81,950	86,048	90,145	94,143	98,340
Nov	62,457	65,580	68,703	71,826	74,948
Dec	67,525	70,901	74,278	77,654	81,030

Okay, let's take this in. In January of last year, you deposited $66,327 with a staff of 5 people. With a 5% increase of deposits to $69,643, you will give each one of those staff $100. Do the math.

- You deposited $3,316 more in that month than you did in the same time period last year.
- You paid out $500 in bonuses.
- The net for you is $2,816.

Let's say that in that same month you have killer growth and increase your deposits by 20%. Do the math.

- You deposited $13,265 more in that month than you did in the same time period last year.
- You paid out $875 in bonuses.
- The net for you is $12,390.

This is a win/win for you. When your month is chugging along, and you know that if your staff works just a little bit harder filling the schedule or they need a little motivation to sell frames or contacts, this is how you get them to where they need to be.

This is also where your projections come into place. If your staff is aware of these numbers and they know how to project, they motivate themselves. But your input and your awareness of the numbers always helps as well.

For example, if it is day 15 out of 20 in the month, and the staff see that they are falling a bit short of receiving their 5% bonus, then they know that with a little extra effort, they can hit their numbers. I mean, what else is going to motivate them? If you have two business days left to go, or even just one, what is going to motivate your staff to pack their Friday schedule? Nothing really. In fact, without something like this in place, you'll notice your Friday schedules becoming more and more light. Your encouragement to them with a desire to pay them their bonus helps them work harder.

I have seen this exact scenario take place. One time, I was at an office on a Friday morning. I knew that there were several openings in the afternoon. Two patients called in a row asking about available exams, and the response they received was that there were openings next week. I thought, "What about today?"

Well, without some motivation to hit a number like a deposit, I'm afraid people are going to default to what is easiest. But if the staff is working towards getting $100, those two phone calls will be a blessing (and worth somewhere around $600). If you don't see this motivating your staff, you probably need new staff.

Photo Bonus

Not every office has a camera taking routine photos, but they have become the standard of care. Some offices just build those photos into their exam which is fine, but you are not being reimbursed for those by most insurance companies. So many practices offer a routine photo for diagnostic purposes at an extra cost of anywhere from $25 to $50.

Spending money above and beyond a copay is understandably not an easy thing to convince a patient to do. But the photo gives you as a doctor real, helpful information about your patient's ocular health. Motivating your workup person to ask your patients for this additional service is not an easy thing to do. So spiff them to motivate them.

Look at your averages over the last year, create a chart much like the deposit chart with projected % improvements, and spiff them. Very little else will get your tech to go above and beyond their normal patterns and areas of comfortability. Imagine spiffing your tech $50 after they sell 25 more photos than last month at $25 a pop. The math is easy. You deposited $1,250, spiffed $50, netted $1,200, and your patients received more comprehensive eye care.

One last note on camera spiffs. It might help your techs if you give them a script to memorize and adapt at first. They just flat out may need the help. Here is one that you can adapt as needed.

"Retinal photographs are the standard of care chosen by Drs. _____ and _____ because they serve as a baseline for your ocular health. The Drs. recommend that all first time patients get them. Additional photos are only necessary when the Drs. feel that there is an issue to monitor. Despite the value of these photos, your insurance does not cover their cost, so there is an additional charge of $25. Can we take those photos for you today?"

Of course, your tech can customize this script once they grow comfortable with it, but getting them started with something like this is typically a big help.

Year's Supply of Contact Lens

At all times, you should know the % of your patients that are contact lens wearers. The easy way to do that is to walk through each month of last year and divide the number of contact lens evaluations by the total number of comprehensive eye exams. Most docs run somewhere between 25% - 33%, but I do know a few that are a bit higher.

Once you know that number, you should be able to set realistic expectations for how many years' supplies of contacts you want to sell each month. Put that in front of your front desk and techs, and spiff them if they hit that number. An organized, motivated mindset to sell a year's supply will definitively increase sells. I saw this demonstrated back in the gravy days. Let me explain.

Many years ago, back when sales reps could directly spiff docs for selling their products, we had a contact lens rep cut a deal with us. If we sold 200 year's supply of their brand of contacts in a 3 month period, the rep would take the entire staff to Ruth Chris steakhouse. In essence, the rep was offering to pay for 18 people to eat whatever they wanted at an incredibly high end restaurant if we pushed her contacts. Now of course, these types of practices are illegal these days, but guess what happened back then? We sold 200 year's supplies of her contact in 8 weeks…and the steak was very good; thank you very much. All it took was some motivation.

Now this is a good time to talk about retaining contact lens sells, so let me speak to that for a second. This issue is much like the issue in facing the big box stores. You cannot compete with 1-800-get your contacts cheap or the big box stores. Now, you can negotiate contact lens prices, and you should let your contact lens rep know that for the most part, they are all the same. You don't tell your patients that, but the differences aren't more than minimal.

Bottom line: if your rep doesn't negotiate, tell them you are finding a new lens or a new rep.

But back to retaining your contacts lens sells. You, your front desk, and your techs have got to be on the same page when it comes to selling contacts. You are always going to offer your patients your best deal by selling year's supplies.

Now, I know in this economy, dropping $180 - $250 dollars at a time for contacts is a tough pill to swallow. But you have got to explain to your patients that this is their best deal. They will either nickel and dime it online and pay exorbitant shipping and handling or they can find a healthy price with you. Negotiate with your vendors. Some of them will ship directly to the patients with no cost. And you know what? 1-800-whatever is not going to replace a bad contact if you get one. You will. Your folks have got to make this effort.

Now, I know some docs who tell me that their patients buy all their contacts from them anyway, they just don't buy a year's supply at one time. Their patients call in 3-4 times a year, so there is no need to push it. If that is your situation, good for you, but there is one problem with that scenario. You are losing money. Let me explain.

Let's say your patient gets contacts from you 4 times a year: at their yearly exam, and every 3 months after that. Well, those 3 times that they call in throughout the year cost you money. Your employee answers the phone 3 times, pulls their chart/looks them up on the computer 3 times, orders their contacts 3 times, processes their orders when they come in 3 times, calls your patient back 3 times, and dispenses those contacts 3 times. Yeah, you received your patient's money for a year supply, but you wound up making a lot less money.

Maybe each of those interactions took 3 minutes of your employee's time. That employee makes $10 an hour. 3 minutes is worth $.50. Since your patient keeps calling in, you paid your employee $3.00 to process all of those orders which made your already thin profit on contacts even smaller.

Bottom Line: Teach your staff to sell year's supplies.

Insurance Bonus

Most doctors do not manage their insurance person because they just don't know the inner workings of insurance. Additionally, I've known OD's who have kept horrible insurance people around because they just assumed that they couldn't find another and they feared what would happen income-wise if they didn't have someone in that spot for 2 weeks. Don't do that. **Fire bad employees.**

Losing two weeks of insurance income is probably less than what you are losing by employing an insurance person who is not getting it done.

The good thing about an insurance bonus is that it is a built in accountability module. If they don't hit the numbers, they don't get a bonus, and you have questions to ask. And hear me on this: you must meet face to face with your insurance person each month. So much so, that you are familiar with your insurance balances in each age category (0-30, 31-60, etc). You need to be able to ask about specific outstanding balances.

For example, sometimes getting paid for post-op cataract work is incredibly hard. You might be owed over $400 for a single patient that is over 60 days old. You have got to know this and manage this, and I'll tell you why. I do not mean to impugn your insurance person, but there will always be a temptation to just write off difficult claims so as not to have too high of old balances. And in the big picture, if you are not managing these things, you will never know it. $400 in your write off total will probably not even be noticed. So here is how you spiff/manage your insurance person.

I suggest giving your insurance person $100 - $150 if all of their insurance totals 90 days and under are 97% or higher of their overall outstanding insurance. I know that sounds convoluted, so let me explain.

With this plan, only 3% of your entire outstanding insurance total is 91 days or older. 90 days is plenty of time for a claim to filed, fixed, and re-filed. A good insurance person can even get 3 filings in in 90 days. Any claim over 90 days is definitively in jeopardy of being collected, and your person has got to know what the issue is by that time. The formula for determining these numbers is as follows:

Current + (31–60) + (61-90) divided by insurance **total**

For example, let's say these are your outstanding insurance numbers.

(Current) $28,758.03 + **(31-60)** $1973.77 + **(61-90)** $366.79 = $31,098.59

Your Total Outstanding Insurance = $32,484.59

(All Insurance 90 days and Younger) $31,098.59 divided by **(Your Total Outstanding Insurance)** $32,484.59 = .957 or 96%

In this scenario, your insurance person would not receive a bonus for the month. The best idea is to get your numbers presently, plug them in, and find out the health of your outstanding Insurance A/R. As soon as you do this, you are probably going to realize that implementing a plan like this is going to require a massive cleanup of your outstanding insurance.

Sit down with your insurance person and speak about every single over 90 claim and any 61-90 day claim (as they will be over 90 very soon). You might be surprised to find out that you have claims on the books that are years old. More than likely, you aren't ever going to collect them, and you will just have to write them off. Claims that are a year old, or are otherwise seen as uncollectable, just have to go off the books.

Clean the numbers up, and start your insurance person off with some of hitting their goal. But your insurance person can only write off the claims that you approve. They can still pursue them if they feel they are possibly going to collect them in the future, but this will be gut-check time for both of you. Your writing some claims off is going to hurt, but they weren't coming in anyway. Doing this shows your insurance person that you are going to help them move towards hitting this number on a regular basis.

You might consider moving it to 5% of over 90 (which is completely up to you) or you might want to change it over a few months. Spiff your person on 5% for the first 3-6 months knowing that it will be spiffed off of 3% going forward. You'll find your insurance person fighting harder for claims, they will keep a better check on your front desk to make sure they are verifying insurance, and you will collect a higher % of your claims and deposit more money.

Optical Bonus

The first and most important optical bonus you can implement is when your sellers move a number of frames consistent with your goals. For example, if you want to turn your frame board over 2.5 times a year, then figure out the number of frames that have to be sold in a year. Divide that by the weeks you are open and even go so far as to break down by day.

Understandably, your office more than likely closes for Thanksgiving and Christmas and Easter, so just go ahead and set your weeks of operation at 50. Let's use an office with 400 frames on the frame board for our example.

600 frames x 2.5 = 1,500 projected frames sold a year
1,500 frames divided by 50 weeks = 30 frames sold a week.
30 frames a week divided by 5 business days = 6 frames a day.

Now before we talk about spiffing these numbers, your first reaction might be, "What? I better sell more than 6 frames a day." First of all this is just a hypothetical, and secondly, and I hate to do this to you, check and see how many frames you sold last year.

Add up the total, divide by 250, and you'll probably be shocked. I hope not, but chances are you might be.

Either way, let's use these numbers for our examples: 30 frames a week and 6 a day. First of all, if your optical hits 30 a week, bonus them. Figure out the best number, but let's say you give your sellers $50 each week they hit their number. Don't panic; you are paying out $100 in bonuses (to two staff) only and if they sell 30 frames. The average frame price is probably $179 or so. Do the math. They sell $5,370 worth of frames and you pay out $100. It will be okay. The important thing is you want your sellers motivated.

I used to spiff my optical daily. Seriously. I would even let the benefits spread to the whole office. It worked like this. If the staff hit their daily numbers, I would buy the office breakfast. Or I would tier it; sell 2 more frames than your daily total, and everyone gets muffins!

Before you think that I went broke buying muffins, stop worrying. It always paid out. The staff had a couple of cheap options for breakfast. Typically it was donuts or muffins. So let's say my optical sold 8 frames one day. Average frame price was $179 so we sold $1,432 worth of frames. I would then spend $12 on muffins for the whole staff. Everyone was motivated, and everyone was fed. The steady (and increased sales) always made the cost of food worth it.

I have seen my staff absolutely kill themselves and then celebrate to get that last frame sale at the end of the day just so they could get muffins. I loved it. I encouraged it. Every day, I would walk in the office, verify the deposit, check to see if they hit their numbers, and then head out on my errands. I would make the deposit, and then I would pick up donuts for everyone. Life was good on those days.

Weekly Bonus

Weekly bonuses work the same way, of course. You need to sell your 30 frames per week, and you need to find a way to spiff your staff. Again, I encourage an all office spiff. Pick 4-5 affordable restaurants around you and make lunch the spiff. A great way to start a Monday is eating the lunch earned on Friday. And again, the cost is no big deal. Pizza, subs, etc are going to run you $50 or so for lunch. Your staff sold $5,370 worth of frames (30 x $179 avg frame price). In the long run, if your staff is consistently turning over their frame boards, $50 worth of pizza is no big deal.

An added bonus is that sharing the spiff with the whole staff will improve inter-office relations. No matter how hard you have worked to protect salary anonymity, your staff assumes the frame sellers make more money. I've seen this turn really ugly before. The front desk person who gets to eat subs because the frame sellers did their job well has one less thing to complain about.

Spiffing Your Front Desk

The most effective spiff for your front desk is how full they keep your schedule. For this to have its largest impact on your bottom line, you are going to have to monitor it well. Let me explain.

I recommend a spiff based on a % of your schedule being filled. For example, if you are a practice with a healthy patient base, you may be scheduled out for a week or so at the time. That is a great problem to have, and you want to address that problem by seeing as many comprehensive eye exams in one day as you can. So, pick a % that is going to make your staff work hard and efficiently. For sake of demonstration, I'm going to choose 95% as the goal. You can choose whatever you think will make your staff work hard but also be reachable.

To get to 95%, several things need to be in place. First and foremost, there has to be a schedule template. Staff must be instructed as to where and when they place exams, office visits, and follow ups on your schedule. Never leave it to the whims of your front desk person. Though they may mean well, without motivation and accountability, your staff is always going to schedule your staff as to what is convenient for them. Without a template, you will almost never have a full schedule at the end of a day, and I guarantee you that you won't have busy schedules on Friday afternoons.

Your job is to tell the front desk where and when to schedule; their job is to fill that schedule.

There are as many sample templates as there are OD's in this world, so I offer one merely to get you to examine your day and make the determination for yourself. To begin, ask yourself this question, "How many comprehensive eye exams can I see in one uninterrupted hour?" I've seen one doctor choose anywhere between 1 and 6. For the sake of this discussion, let's go with 3.

Now look at when you start your day, when you go to lunch, and when you want to leave. The first 20 minutes of your day should be follow up and medical exams. The 20 minutes prior to lunch should be the same, the first 20 minutes after lunch, and the final 20 minutes of your day should be the same. With 10 minutes for each appointment, you have 8 slots each day to see follow ups and sick-eyes. That is plenty. The rest of the day should be reserved for comprehensive exams which offer you your greatest opportunity for revenue.

Let's say you open your doors at 8:00am and close at 5:00. You take lunch from 12:00pm to 1:00 pm. Then your template looks like this:

Time	Appointment
8:00 am	Follow Up/Sick Eye
8:10 am	Follow Up/Sick Eye
8:20 am	Comprehensive Exam
8:40 am	Comprehensive Exam
9:00 am	Comprehensive Exam
9:20 am	Comprehensive Exam
9:40 am	Comprehensive Exam
10:00 am	Comprehensive Exam
10:20 am	Comprehensive Exam
10:40 am	Comprehensive Exam
11:00 am	Comprehensive Exam
11:20 am	Comprehensive Exam

11:40 am	Follow Up/Sick Eye
11:50 am	Follow Up/Sick Eye
12:00 pm	Lunch
1:00 pm	Follow Up/Sick Eye
1:10 pm	Follow Up/Sick Eye
1:20 pm	Comprehensive Exam
1:40 pm	Comprehensive Exam
2:00 pm	Comprehensive Exam
2:20 pm	Comprehensive Exam
2:40 pm	Comprehensive Exam
3:00 pm	Comprehensive Exam
3:20 pm	Comprehensive Exam
3:40 pm	Comprehensive Exam
4:00 pm	Comprehensive Exam
4:20 pm	Comprehensive Exam
4:40 pm	Follow Up/Sick Eye
5:00 pm	Follow Up/Sick Eye

With this schedule, you can see 20 comprehensive exams a day and 8 follow ups and sick eyes. Now, that may look like a sweet schedule, but recognize that in a typical 20 business day month, you would see 400 comprehensive exams. That would be sweet if you have the patient base. If you feel that number is one you would have to grow into, then adjust your schedule to 2 full exams and hour (depending upon where you start and start, that would give you 13-15 exams a day and 260-300 exams a month).

Okay, spiffs for your front desk can be made up of a various items, but I like to go food for weekly and money for monthly. If 95% occupancy is your goal on a 3 exams an hour schedule, then the entire office gets lunch if you see 95 exams during the week. If you already have a lunch scheduled for Monday because of optical, great, then the staff gets lunch Monday and Tuesday. A monthly spiff is easy to come up with; just remind yourself of the additional income you are enjoying because of the fuller schedule.

A Simple Effective Marketing Plan

Even the best of offices need to do marketing. Folks move so much these days, and those new to your neighborhood need to know where to find eye care. Well, first and foremost, do the easy thing: get a Facebook page and update it regularly. Advertise at your front desk for your patients to "like" your page. But this next piece of advice is just as important.

Update your page regularly, so you remain in your patient's online consciousness. If you have a million "likes" but never update the page, what good is it? Task your optical to give you at least two updates a week. Task your front desk to give you at least one. Then, you make sure you are speaking about ocular health once a week. It is easy, it is free, and it is effective.

But to find new folks, you might just have to do a postcard effort. Normally, an effective by-mail marketing campaign requires at least a 10,000 piece mailer. They look something like this.

- 10,000 postcards mailed to roughly 3,300 homes, 3 separate times over the course of a month
- The drawback to these types of mailers is that they often cost between $4,000 - $5,000 and all of that cost is up front.
- In addition, these types of efforts take $8,000 - $10,000 in gained revenue to justify the expense.

So, an alternative is a precision marketing mailing campaign to a predominantly new or strategically located neighborhood coupled with customized web marketing. Here is what the process would look like.

- Choose a 300-500 home, new-construction community within a mile or two of your office.

Since these are all homes located near your office, the owners are looking for convenience and accessibility. The neighborhood is new, so the owners are open to new services and service providers.

- The next step is to send 3 mailers to each home over the course of a month.

However, sending 3 separate mailers to these homes is still not enough to make the campaign effective. Incentive and target marketing are necessary. Each postcard should include both a map to your location and discount of some sort when the recipient brings in the postcard.

- But the key to this whole effort is the internet target marketing.

Included on the flier is an alias/ghost website address with the neighborhood's name in it (www.eyedrforneighborhood.com) pointing to a customized page on your office site that details how your office can care for that neighborhood. A webpage with the community name in it coupled with 3 mailers and a % off incentive will greatly increase the effectiveness of the campaign. Be sure to include a "like us on Facebook/follow us on Twitter" note as well.

What is the cost?

The cost of the design is dependent upon whether you have material ready or not, but most designers would not charge more than $150.

- 1,500 postcards are roughly $300 (that includes the printing at www.vistaprint.com).
- The website url is $10.
- The postage is $400 or less
- Essentially, you have an effective marketing campaign for well under $1,000

But you ask, "Where do I get the addresses?" That is typically what you are paying for with a marketing company. Do this: check your county's tax records online. Most post them for free right now. Task someone in your office to compile those addresses or pay your kid $25 to do it for you at night. The info is there. You don't have to pay a company to get it for you.

Appendix

As we wrap these thoughts on increasing revenue I thought it would be helpful to just include a couple sample forms that I have found useful over the years.

Feel free to print them up and use them as you will. Feel free to manipulate them in any way that you see helpful. Bottom line: always lead your staff where you want them to go. There are a few resourceful employees left out that, but most of them to be directed and directed specifically.

So towards that end what you'll find are a few handouts that have been helpful over the years. Included are:

- The process for transferring balances from insurances to patients.
- Insurance pre-authorization forms.
- Notes to patients who have been absent for a long period of time.
- Sample employee evaluations.

Insurance Balance Transfer Policy

Responsible Parties: _____

- At the end of each day, the staff person at check out will search the end of the day report for any insurance balances transferred to a patient.
- They will highlight, note, or explain the balance transfer giving further detail on the transfer offering to answer any questions related to the new balance.
- Notify _____ of each before mailing them out.
- Once approved, drop them in the mail.
- This process is unnecessary the five business days prior to the 26th so as not to annoy patients with two mailers in one.
- All statements that are printed on the 26th should be highlighted and have personal notes.
- Begin the process again with any transfers from the 27th on.

Patient Pre-Authorization

- Patient Name:

- Date of Appointment:

- DOB:

- SS #:

- Insurance:

- Insurance ID:

- Guarantor (if different than patient):

- Insurance Verification:

- SW & Date:

- Pre-Authorization # or Date of Eligibility:

Lost Patient Letter

Dear Patient,

During an overview of our records, we made a startling discovery: We have not had the privilege of caring for you or your eyes in over 3 years. Lots of reasons contribute to missing an eye exam, but we want to make sure you know that we value you and the health of your eyes.

Knowing that everyone's schedules are busy and times are hard, we want to give you an incentive to come in for an eye exam. Just make an appointment, bring in this card, and you will receive either free single vision or bifocal lenses with the purchase of a frame.

This is our way of showing how much we appreciate you. If you have any questions or would like to make an appointment, please call_____.

Employee Review

**Rank Yourself in the
Following categories from 1-5
1 is the lowest and 5 is the highest
With each category, include an explanation**

EMPLOYEE NAME:
SIGNATURE:

1. Punctuality: _____

    Explain:

2. Appearance: _____

    Explain:

3. Job Knowledge: _____

    Explain:

4. Efficiency: _____

    Explain:

5. Accuracy: _____

    Explain:

6. Dependability: _____

    Explain:

7. Innovativeness: _____

    Explain:

8. Professionalism: _____

    Explain:

9. Patient Interaction: _____

    Explain:

10. Leadership: _____

    Explain:

11. Staff Relations: _____

    Explain:

One Final Note:

Thank you so much for taking the time to read this book. It has been born out of a million mistakes, and I hope that it enables you to avoid the ones confessed to here. As an old mentor use to say, "Mistakes are okay. Just make brand new one and avoid the old ones."

If there is ever any way in which I can help you or refer you to other resources, don't hesitate to contact me. You can always find more information at www.practiceprogress.com or at our Facebook page.

You can always email me at gordon@practiceprogress.com.